Helping People Stay Fit While Earning A Side Income

BY

I0695891

Lovely

Copyright © 2020

Disclaimer

All the material contained in this book is provided for educational and informational purposes only. No responsibility can be taken for any results or outcomes resulting from the use of this material.

While every attempt has been made to provide information that is both accurate and effective, the author does not assume any responsibility for the accuracy or use/misuse of this information.

INTRODUCTION

The fitness industry is one of the most lucrative industries in the world. It's also extremely competitive, with countless people attempting to break into it.

As a result, you may be wondering how to make money with fitness.

Many people are turning to trained professionals such as trainers, instructors, and coaches as they become more conscious of their health and physical activity levels.

And, as with any in-demand profession, there are numerous ways to monetize your skillset, whether through offering services or developing products. As a side hustle, we could lead a workout class.

A 'side hustle' is a term commonly used to describe an additional job that can be done in addition to a primary source of income, with many people preferring to work on a part-time, or zero-hour, basis.

The reasons for this decision can range from financial gain to personal fulfillment, and are often unique to an individual.

For example, if you've always wanted to be a part-time personal trainer, this side hustle can help you get there while also providing job satisfaction and a higher rate of pay.

In reference to the definition of a side hustle provided above, I consider myself a side hustle queen because I've tried several side hustles over the years while raising three children as a single mother.

You may be wondering how trying various side hustles over the years qualifies me as a Side Hustle Queen.

So, here's my story!

I'd always worked as an employee, but I knew deep down that I wasn't cut out for working for someone else. I recall being fourteen years old and receiving my first paycheck. I worked in fast food and was startled at how little I was paid, so I began stealing from them.

It wasn't much, maybe a $20 bill every few days, and only when I felt confident I could get away with it.

The irony is that I volunteered at a different store one day and was accused of stealing from their register when I was completely innocent. To be honest, it scared me and caused me to stop. I subsequently discovered that one of the employees would steal from the new person's register and get them in trouble. That day, I was a newcomer. All of this is to say that when I was 14, I realized I wanted to be an entrepreneur and also wanted to get rich quickly. I've also fallen for a few pyramid schemes throughout the years. The first was Avon. I'd get boxes of items every two weeks and even hired individuals to work for me. What they didn't tell me was that you had to spend your profit on catalogs, logo receipts, logo bags, samples, and everything else, Avon.

They also omitted to disclose that you will not receive a check. So you pay up ahead, get the goods, and keep whatever money you make. Avon is not the only corporation that operates in this manner. Maybe I didn't do it correctly, or maybe these kinds of setups are designed to make the firms rich while keeping us hoping. Please keep in mind that I did not learn my lesson. I literally bought into the flower pyramid scheme. You know, the one where you pay the person in the heart of the flower fifty bucks to have your name engraved on a flower petal? The team then works hard to convince new people to join them. Your name gets moved closer and closer to the center as they buy in your name, and once you reach the center, BOOM! You are compensated. I never made it to the heart of the matter.

I opened a restaurant when I was 26 years old. It was so busy that I had to arrange a food truck as well. Yes, my wish had been granted! I also divorced when I was 25, becoming a single mother of three children. So there I was, a local celebrity as a result of my restaurant's popularity, with so many customers that I couldn't keep up. No, seriously! I was unable to keep up. I began asking for free assistance from friends and relatives. I had a fantastic support system but no good help, so I began hiring individuals. I quickly discovered that no one wants to work for minimum wage, especially if the work is difficult, and the restaurant sector is difficult! I had been operating for seven years when I decided to sell everything and relocate to another state.

For me, starting anew was a positive thing. Not materially but psychologically. I was stressed out from attempting to run a restaurant on my own, and I had bought a couple of residences. Aside from everything else, I was also trying to be a landlord, although I was seven hundred miles away. That didn't work either. This was before Airbnb and low-cost property management became popular.

I found work as soon as I arrived in my new city. It was straightforward, adequately paid, and exactly what I needed until one morning when I awoke with a severe cramp in my hand. It began with the left hand but swiftly moved to the right. When I was finally able to see my doctor, she diagnosed me with severe carpal tunnel syndrome. Now, I'd heard of several people experiencing this, and there was no way it could be that severe. It certainly was for me! I had two unsuccessful procedures in a row. To no avail, I went through rehab, therapy, and all other procedures that the doctors prescribed. I even took steroids and acquired a lot of extra weight for nothing.

I'm still suffering from carpal tunnel syndrome. I had to not only abandon my career but also find something that didn't place too much strain on my hands. Nothing paid well enough to sustain three children, so I had to work extra hours. I've tried so many different side hustles. Some were successful, while others were not, but keep reading, and I'll reveal how I became a side hustle queen.

I recall staying up all night worrying about how I was going to feed my children and whether I would be able to pay my rent. I would wonder if I made a bad decision in starting over and moving so far from my family, and I would regret selling my houses and restaurant. I would think *no matter how much work they were, I had income.*

You may probably tell from my introduction that I am a lady of action. I began by conducting research. During those sleepless evenings, I would watch YouTube videos and read books and articles. The majority of people said the same thing and recommended the same side hustles. I thoroughly tested them all well, as many as I could. If everyone is telling you to do the same thing, there must be money to be made, right? Wrong! Some of them were OK, but many of them were and are saturated, or their time has passed.

I needed to be creative, so I attempted numerous side hustles throughout the years. Now, I'm going to share with you one of the side hustles that I can comfortably employ to support myself and my family. This side hustle book leading a workout class is one of several side hustles I intend to write or have already written. Please keep in mind that everything I'll be presenting here is based on my own experiences and research throughout the years. It worked for me, but not everything works for everyone. So, if this does not work for you, you can look through my other volumes on side hustles to see which ones would.

If you're less than happy in your 9-5 job, then a fitness side hustle can help you to maintain your current role whilst allowing you to do what you really love doing. In the case of a personal trainer, yoga, Pilates or exercise to music instructor, that would be helping people by creating and delivering great fitness training sessions. A side hustle can help bridge the gap between what you want to do and what you need to do.

In this book, we'll take an in-depth look at how you can make money in the fitness industry while still keeping your full time job and doing what you love.

So if you're ready to get started on this lucrative journey toward financial freedom, let's get moving!

BENEFITS OF FITNESS SIDE HUSTLE

If you're young and enjoy exercise, I think becoming a fitness instructor is one of the best side hustles out there – it pushes you, it's humbling, it requires you to energetically lead a room, and it's actually pretty fantastic for getting to know new people.

I feel compelled to state that it's not for everyone: Merely liking exercise is not enough of a prerequisite for becoming a fitness instructor (which actually involves more theatrics and stamina than actual love of exercise, in my opinion), but I think anyone can be developed to the point where they're pretty good. Therefore, I'll be sharing the benefits of leading a fitness class as a side hustle.

Have a Positive Impact on People's Lives

In your current job you may not feel like you have much of a positive impact on anyone's life. Perhaps you aren't creating the change in the world you'd hoped to. Speak to any personal trainer or fitness professional and they'll tell you one of the greatest rewards of the role is helping people achieve their goals and seeing the positive impact training has on their clients lives. Delivering exercise sessions before and after your regular 9-5 job is a great way to achieve the satisfaction you crave. Regardless of whether you deliver in-person sessions or virtual ones, seeing your clients progress, lose weight, gain muscle or achieve any of their fitness related goals gives you a feeling you won't get in a regular/non-fitness job.

There's a Social Up-side to the Fitness Side Hustle

The fitness industry is one of the most social industries there is, while for many people, their 9-5 doesn't give them the social atmosphere they really enjoy. Coaching fitness is a person-to-person activity, you have to be social. Not only does being social help you, but also helps your clients achieve their goals and improve their overall wellbeing. A study on the effects of physical activity on social interactions showed those that exercise have more trust and are prone to more "prosocial" behaviors than those that don't. If you are a social creature, then the fitness side-hustle will not only help you see improvements in someone's fitness, but also in other aspects of their life as well.

Adds Variety to Your Life

If your day to day is filled with the "same-old-same-old", offering a variety of fitness services in your side hustle is a great way to spice things up. Whether it be a one-to-one workout using body weight, a yoga or Pilates class, or even a T3 HIIT workout, the variety of workouts you can offer is limited only by your qualification and skills. Your clients will also benefit from different types of training, and they'll appreciate the variety as well.

You Choose When You Side Hustle

This benefit is true for all fitness professionals regardless of whether they're doing it full or part time. When working in fitness, you have a lot more flexibility in choosing when you work and when you don't. You can decide when you train clients or deliver your classes, which makes it easier to fit the rest of your private life in and around your career.

If you only want to earn a little, then you can just have a couple of clients. Or if you're saving up for your next big purchase, you can take on more clients and classes as your time permits.

You Can Do It All From Home

The COVID-19 pandemic has made virtual training sessions the norm. Analysts believe the virtual fitness market will continue to grow over the coming years, hitting a global market value of over £49 billion by

2027. Research has also shown that many clients expect to incorporate virtual training into their regular schedule when things "return to normal". Offering a virtual fitness side hustle will allow you to maximize your time, as you don't have to travel to a gym, and allow you to keep everything you earn as there is no fee to pay the gym. If you teach group classes as well, you get to keep the fees you charge from each participant, making the more the merrier. Virtual is definitely the way to go.

A Great Earning Potential

A good side hustle should ultimately lead to additional income. Even if money isn't your main motivation, you should still charge for your services, time and efforts. If you're not sure what to charge, shop around and see what others in your area are charging.

BECOME A GROUP FITNESS INSTRUCTOR

Fitness has become really big since the 80's. There has been a rise in yoga, aerobics and weightlifting. People have become serious about their health and rightly so. I'm not sure if it's been your dream to own a yoga or dance studio but that is not what I mean. I'm suggesting something a little more meek like $5/week for a group workout in the park on Saturday mornings.

I know that anyone can go for a walk in the park so you'll have to make it interesting. For example bring a Bluetooth speaker and walk to all Christian music or Michael Jackson songs. Your walks can be themed I.E. everyone wears a certain color or some of the proceeds go to a charity. The possibilities are endless!

It could be something as simple as you lead stretches before and after. People are going to participate not only for the fitness aspect but also for the fellowship. We like to belong to something and we love to talk about the good things we are doing in our lives.

While I am not the end-all of career advice and everyone has a different situation, I wanted to share some of the general tips that worked for me.

How to Become a Group Fitness Instructor

Find out what you like and identify your favorite program and specialty.

When you feel like you have the desire to stand at the front of the group fitness room and lead, you have to make sure you are passionate about what you will be teaching. The first thing you should do is find a class or group fitness program that you absolutely love, whether that's yoga, cardio bootcamp or even dance fitness. Become a regular in that class and learn the ins and outs of taking the class like the back of your hand. That's your first step. Identify your program/form of movement of choice and become a skilled student in that format. Rather than saying you want to teach anything, choose one thing and study it deeply.

Consider learning a pre-choreographed program to start.

I would definitely recommend that your entrance to teaching group fitness come in the form of learning to teach a pre-choreographed program like Zumba, Turbo Kick, etc. because that means you can take "have to program and come up with sound movements and music" out of the equation when you are just beginning your career in fitness. Many times you can get certified to teach these pre-choreographed programs without any previous fitness experience, because all you will be doing is delivering the workout to people in a group fitness studio, and the experts with the fitness background have made up the moves and programming for you ahead of time.

You can go to each of the individual pre-choreographed group fitness program websites to see what it takes to become an instructor and most require an in-person training weekend, followed by submitting a video of you teaching a full class after the fact, with ongoing education required.

Speak to your group fitness instructor, and connect with the group fitness manager of your gym or studio.

At larger box gyms there is usually a group fitness manager, with whom you may never cross paths. Oftentimes you can find out that person's email address by asking at the front desk of the gym (or looking on the top or back of a printed group fitness schedule). And at smaller studios, you may be able to talk to the studio manager just by going up to the desk. You absolutely want to communicate with this person and begin to build a relationship. No need to be embarrassed at all, in fact, they will be happy to chat with you, get to know you, and then they will be able to help you along your journey. Also, most importantly, let your group fitness instructor know that you are interested in learning to teach.

The GFM (group fitness manager) and studio manager (SM), will be able to tell you if there are upcoming trainings or opportunities in the near future and keep you in mind. They may also tell you what you need to do to work toward attending a training or being considered as a trainee (some studios train people in-house and don't require experience, and you want to be first in line for that.

Make your intentions clear with your full-time job, and commit to a regular class schedule.

You will have to find out whether early morning or evening works best for your workload and life and stick to it. The good news is that weekend classes are always up for grabs and rarely get in the way, so consider those as well.

However, you must prepare yourself for some resentment from your full-time employer. While they may be happy that you have an interest in your health, they may soon grow tired of you running out the door to teach classes, especially if it's multiple times a week. I hope you don't experience that, I just need you to be aware it may create some tension when you show commitment to a "hobby" that takes you away from your day job. And also remember that taking on group fitness will require you to say no to other things. When you commit to teaching a regular class, you can't get a sub just because you don't feel like going or have other errands to run or a social activity. That's not how it works.

Prepare to keep learning and investing in new certifications.

When you start teaching group fitness, your fitness journey is really just beginning. Even though you may choose to keep your full-time job in another industry, you will want to keep learning and investing in your fitness education every single day. That means considering whether you want to get general group fitness certifications like an ACE or AFAA group fitness certificate (which requires testing, a workshop, etc.) to grow your knowledge and get extra backing and credentials. You will want to attend continuing education events, like Les Mills advanced instructor modules, or fitness events like the IDEA World Fitness Convention. Or perhaps you want to start studying the science of movement and the body even further and get a personal trainer certification (which is pretty time intensive, but well worth it for what you learn). You'll have to keep practicing your craft, learning more, connecting with other fitness professionals and becoming a better instructor every time you teach a class. The work is just beginning, and that's what makes it so fun.

CREATE AN OUTDOOR GROUP FITNESS CLASS

Outdoor group fitness participation increased dramatically during the pandemic and is still riding a wave of popularity. Have you noticed all the new outdoor-specific equipment and education companies? Perhaps you've already taken advantage of new tools and resources specifically geared for instructors who want to teach outside. Regardless, the outdoor environment can be a bit more complicated than the studio setting. Let's explore the necessary considerations, planning and programming elements of teaching an outdoor class.

Outdoor Group Fitness Considerations

Teaching outdoors may seem more accessible, open and rules-barred, but it can quickly get complicated. I'll be sharing my lessons over the years leading an outdoor group fitness in this section.

Personal Passion

Before reviewing some of the finer points of programming an outdoor group fitness class, it's important to consider whether it's something *you* really want to do. Recognize within yourself that it takes more work and time to teach outdoors. When you're teaching outside, you don't have the luxury of easily accessible equipment, a sound system setup (this is why I recommend a Bluetooth speaker) and a prepared space.

You need to factor in a lot of time for setting up and taking down. You must be willing to show up early, stay afterward and be nimble when things change at the last minute. Don't do it if you're not particularly creative or excited about the outdoor environment.

Scheduling

When it comes to scheduling, most outdoor group fitness classes will be most successful before work, at lunchtime, after work and after school (as with indoor classes). However, the pandemic did make for flexibility in many work schedules, so it may be worth asking participants if they can make it earlier in the day so you don't end up in the dark when the seasons change. The time of day will also affect your given location.

Weather Conditions

The pandemic proved that outdoor classes could be successful year-round in even some of the most unexpected places. While you might think extreme temperatures, wind and rain would prevent participation in colder months, there are plenty of people who are not deterred. In fact, they find community in the misery of discomfort and being in it together However, those who live in areas that are warmer throughout the year may be less interested in going outside when it's colder or raining.

In southern California, people would still be wearing gloves and beanies in the 40s. Everyone's tolerance level is different, which is why you need to be flexible. Rather than complain about the weather, it's crucial to find the silver lining for participants to keep their spirits and energy levels up.

Programming

While this may seem obvious, aim to make your outdoor group fitness classes specific to the outdoors. At this point, we should be making outdoor experiences about the joy of being outside and taking advantage of what an outdoor space has to offer over an indoor space. We aren't working out outside because we have to; we're working out outside because we *want* to, and we're taking full advantage of the space and freedom it offers.

Let's review some outdoor format options, specific outdoor considerations for each, and how you can use the unique elements of the outdoor environment to enhance the experience.

- **Yoga:** Find the flattest location possible. The grass may seem friendly, but bumps and grooves make some poses, especially balancing postures, more challenging. Use cues that highlight the fact that you're outside. For example: "Reach your hands toward the sky;" "Watch the trees swaying while in your tree pose;" "Take a breath of fresh outdoor air;" or "Feel the sun on your face." And create a class plan just for the outdoors: You might offer a long warmup and shorter relaxing poses if it's colder, or teach cooling poses if it's warmer.

- **Sports conditioning:** Educate participants about the value of being exposed to the elements by training outdoors before the big game or event. Choose a large location with plenty of room to sprint, jump and practice agility. Use cones or painted lines for various challenges and games to bring out the competitive spirit in your outdoor athletes.

- **Running:** Teach an outdoor class specific to runners, such as cross-training or leading a running group. Cross-training involves strengthening supporting muscles, refining alignment and teaching mobility exercises, whereas a running group might include a warmup, intervals or long runs, and a cooldown.

- **Cycling:** Similar to running, an outdoor cycling class is a great cross-training opportunity for strengthening strategic muscle groups and improving movement patterns, or it can simply be for a group of cycling enthusiasts who are seeking community and leadership on proper warmup and cooldown exercises and interval/course ideas. You might also create a class that focuses on cycling-specific recovery, with corrective exercises and stretches that target overworked, tight muscles that spend a lot of time in forward flexion.

- **Climbing:** Climbing has seen a significant spike in popularity due, in part, to the rise of indoor climbing gyms. Cross-training for climbing is an excellent option for an outdoor program, especially if you can incorporate suspension training and playground equipment such as monkey bars to develop core and grip strength.

- **Boot camp:** You have so many creative options to choose from when you teach a boot camp class. In addition to using standard (portable) equipment such as resistance bands, suspension trainers, dumbbells and medicine balls, you can also incorporate stairs or bleachers, benches, pullup bars or rings, fences, painted lines, and more.

- **Dance and kickboxing:** While the grass may seem like an ideal place to offer dancing and kickboxing, it can be unpredictable terrain, depending on how freshly cut the grass is, and you never know if or when sprinklers will turn on during class in the early morning or evening hours. When teaching on concrete, remind participants about the increased stress put on the joints, and encourage rest breaks for anyone experiencing

Liability, Logistics and Locations

Whether teaching for a facility or on your own, check the following areas to ensure you're up to date *before* scheduling your first class.

Liability

Check your liability insurance policy. Is it up to date? Does it provide coverage for teaching outdoors? If not, update your coverage.

Make sure your waivers are current. If you're not sure where to begin, reach out to your insurance provider.

Obtain the proper permits. If you plan to teach in a public park or on private property, get permission from the parks and recreation department or the property owner.

Ensure your CPR/AED certifications are up to date.

Visit the space to see if the lighting is adequate and if you'll need to ask permission to turn on additional lighting. Research the crime statistics.

Logistics

Think through the participant experience from beginning to end.

Consider the following questions:

- Where will participants park their cars?
- Where will they put their things (phone, wallet, keys, extra layers of clothing, etc.)?
- How will they sign up for class, and will you track them?
- Will you charge money?
- How will you collect payment?
- How will you communicate changes in location or timing due to weather or other unexpected events?

The answers to these questions largely depend on whether you offer a one-off class or something ongoing. Also, if the weather can be unpredictable in your region, decide if you want a Plan B and how you will communicate updates to participants. One option is to create a group text thread or use WhatsApp or

Facebook Messenger so that you can send last-minute notifications if the location changes or if class is canceled.

Location

Deciding on a location for outdoor fitness can become overly complicated very quickly, so start somewhere! When determining your preferred site, the most critical factors to consider are safety, space, access to bathrooms and parking.

Here's a list of possible locations:

- Park
- Trail
- Field
- Empty lot
- Corporate break areas
- Stadium or sports field
- Playground
- Apartment community center
- Pool deck
- Beach

During the pandemic, many fitness facilities built designated outdoor spaces, often on the grounds of their indoor facility, which is yet another option. Take inventory of *all* your options, and compare pros and cons. Ensure there is enough space for the number of participants you anticipate, and visit these areas on the days and times you're considering, so you can see if other events, landscaping or the sun's location might affect sound, safety, shade, etc.

BECOME A PERSONAL TRAINER

Operating a personal training side hustle has been proven to be both financially and emotionally rewarding. I'm here to explain exactly what you can expect to face within this role.

Furthermore, by engaging with personal training as a side job, you can learn key skills and gain industry experience, while still having the stability of your primary form of employment. This can act as a springboard, allowing you to launch a full-time career in fitness should you so wish.

Things to Consider Before Launching a Personal Training Side Hustle

I can't stress enough how important scheduling is when operating a side hustle. Deciding to take a side job can greatly affect your existing lifestyle, and what was once your downtime will now need to be dedicated to your PT side hustle.

I advise anyone considering taking on this particular role to ensure they have exceptional organizational skills. Without an efficiently planned schedule and ability to stay on top of multiple tasks at once you may quickly burn out, both physically and emotionally.

Schedules can help you differentiate between tasks within your full-time job role and personal trainer side hustle, allowing you to allocate time for each responsibility.

This can include:

- What time you start and finish your full time-job
- When you need to be at the gym training clients
- Deadlines at your full-time job
- Your clients existing goals and training programs

- Reminders for when you need to contact your clients

Therefore, I strongly advise that you take the time to really consider whether your current lifestyle can sustain a side hustle. The roles and responsibilities of a personal trainer can be incredibly demanding at times, a factor which could potentially cause conflict with your full-time employment.

How to Start Your Own Personal Training Side Hustle

Now that you're informed on the circumstances that may surround you prior to entering the fitness industry, we can now discuss how to go about pursuing personal training as a side job.

Get Professionally Qualified

In order to work professionally in the industry as a personal trainer, you need to get qualified.

However, the fitness education sector can be difficult for newcomers to navigate, and you'll want to ensure you get the best certification for your money, one that will teach you about every aspect of personal training.

If you're interested in personal training as a side hustle, it's highly likely you have a fairly busy schedule with full-time employment and other commitments.

Getting professionally qualified is simply a must, and whilst it isn't technically illegal to train without a certification, you won't be able to receive the necessary personal training insurance without one.

Without insurance, you leave yourself open to serious legal issues. For example, if a client is injured or even dies during a session, you could be charged with corporate manslaughter, regardless of whether your routine was safe or not.

So, be sure to start off your personal training side hustle on the right foot and get qualified.

Decide How and Where You're Going to Train Your Clients

Once you've graduated, you will be fully equipped with an array of knowledge relating to personal training.

Following this, you need to decide how you want to put this into practice with your personal training side business. One of the first things you should be asking yourself is how and where you wish to train clients.

However, please remember that you're operating a side business and unfortunately won't have the time to explore the full scope of potential personal training career options that are reserved for your full-time peers.

I have curated a list of careers that are suitable for side-hustles and can easily be accommodated into any busy schedule, including:

- **Contracted roles in gyms** - Popular gym chains are always looking for part-time workers. With this, you'll be required to work a set number of hours per week, and be paid a consistent salary by the gym. This is a great option for a personal trainer side hustle if you're self-employed, work on a very flexible basis, or work a limited number of hours per week. However, if you're already working a full-time job, I'd advise considering other options (like freelancing), as this does come with more significant demands in terms of the hours you'll need to work.

- **Working entirely freelance** - Working on a freelance basis is arguably the best option for those looking to launch a personal training side hustle. This will grant you unlimited scheduling freedom, allowing you to choose the time, location, and clients that you wish to work with.

- **Mobile personal training** - Instead of a client meeting you at a pre-set location, mobile personal trainers will travel to a client. This can be beneficial for those looking to launch a side hustle, as you can keep work local, ensuring that you never waste precious time or energy traveling long distances to meet clients.

- **Online personal training** - The great thing about online personal training is that it can be done wherever and whenever. There are no limitations or constraints, meaning that you can virtually train clients to a schedule that is convenient for you.

Before you begin to create your personal training business plan for this side hustle, you should strive to determine which role will work best for you in the long run.

There may be a number of factors which help to shape and determine your answer such as:

- Availability
- Location
- Personal comfort
- Finances

However, regardless of your circumstance as a personal trainer you should always strive to provide the best possible service to your client. This means playing to your strengths and creating a business plan that is suitable for you.

Research How to Get Clients

When initially launching your personal trainer side hustle you will probably have little to no initial clients. However, in order to ensure your business is sustainable you'll have to learn how to recruit others into your service.

You can attract clients through the following:

- Building a reputation within the wider fitness community
- Building relationships with fellow personal trainers
- Reciprocal marketing
- Social media
- Personal trainer websites
- Email marketing

- Fliers

Please note, all of these methods won't be successful for every single personal trainer. Each individual and business model is unique, meaning that what may work best for some may not work well for you when launching your personal training side hustle.

I would strongly advise attempting multiple of these approaches in order to maximize your potential client base.

From this research, you should be able to determine which methods of client outreach works well for you and your business.

However, I advise all new personal trainers to not feel too disheartened during this process - getting clients is a hard challenge and not something that can just happen overnight.

Take time to research and implement multiple methods and I promise you will be able to reap the rewards.

Design Your Own Pricing Packages

Designing pricing packages can be somewhat of a challenge for even the most advanced and experienced trainers.

Therefore, when starting personal training as a side job it may be wise to keep these designs simple. Over complication will lead to lower closing rates, meaning you will have fewer clients and less money.

Price per session should reduce in price the more sessions per week a client buys, but the exact amount you choose to charge is entirely up to you.

It may be worth researching fellow competitors in the local area in order to get a better sense of what they're providing and charging.

This can help to better inform you on how you should be designing your packages, as you can determine whether you're going to price match them, or charge a higher rate for additional services your competitors don't provide.

As evident from the four points provided above, a lot of time and dedication needs to go into launching a personal training side hustle.

While this may not be your primary source of income you still need to treat it with the same respect as your other forms of employment.

Failure to maintain all of the aforementioned points will simply result in your business failing, meaning that your side hustle will not be as emotionally or financially beneficial as you'd desire.

Tips for Running Your Personal Trainer Side Hustle

Operating as a personal trainer as a side hustle can be challenging, time-consuming, and emotionally taxing. Therefore, I advise following these tips in order to find financial and emotional success.

Identify a Gap in The Market

When deciding to pursue personal training as a side hustle you should be looking for gaps in the existing market. This will ensure you stand out among competitors and will potentially attract more clients to your business.

In order to find these gaps you'll need to do market research, such as Internet searches and discussions with existing personal trainers.

From this, you could discover that your local competitors only offer basic personal training. In this instance, one way to stand out among clients would be to achieve a specialist qualification, such as Lower Back Pain Management

This is considered to be a gap in the market, as you will be able to provide a service that your competitors do not.

If you offer the exact same training as your competitors you'll simply be lost among the crowd, with no defining traits or services to encourage clients to choose you over your competitors.

Therefore, you should always be looking to stand out, even if a competitor does provide a similar or identical service. If this occurs, try to think of an alternative way to approach your training from, in order to find a gap in the market.

Immediately Define Your Goals

When starting a personal training as a side job you need to immediately define your goals, this will help you to determine what you personally want out of the job.

These goals must be specific to you, and can be personable relating to your emotional satisfaction, or they could be profitable and relate to financial satisfaction.

However, these goals shouldn't be too vague as this can lead to personal dissatisfaction and a lack of direction for your business.

An example of a vague goal would be - *"I want to get more clients"*. This is considered directionless, as it doesn't state how many clients the trainer wishes to recruit, nor does it set a timeframe that this goal should be achieved by.

To avoid falling into this pitfall, I'll advise implementing SMART goals throughout your side hustle.

An example of how to apply SMART goals to side hustle would be: *"I want to recruit 3 more clients in 2 months"*

This goal has specifically stated the trainer wishes to recruit a further 3 clients, which can easily be measured, in the time-bound deadline of 2 months. Whether these goals are realistically achievable is dependent on the individual.

When setting these goals you must be realistic and honest with yourself and your own capabilities. Don't set something that is too far out of reach, as this will only lead to disappointment should it not be met.

Compartmentalize Your Side Hustle From Your Current Employment

A personal training side hustle should never interfere with your primary source of employment. Be sure to maintain a meticulous level of organization, in order to ensure that your focus on one role doesn't affect the other.

For example, don't be answering calls, emails and messages regarding training sessions during your full-time working hours. This could lead you to underperforming in your existing role, which could get you into trouble with your employer.

Let your clients know that you have another job that demands your attention during set hours of the day. It will also help to provide a schedule of your availability, ensuring that these clients know when you're available to take their enquiry.

Furthermore, you may also need to inform your current employer that you're running a side hustle, especially if you could be viewed as direct competitors within the fitness industry.

If this is the case there may be a clause in your contract that forbids you to operate in your side hustle role. Should you be found breaching this contract without informing your employer, it could result in legal issues or termination from your existing role.

Therefore, in order to create this defined separation between roles, you absolutely need to ensure that your employer knows what you're doing.

Keep an Accurate Record of All Your Finances

When running a business passion and knowledge can only get you so far. Whilst you may be a fitness expert with a specialist Obesity & Weight Management qualification under your belt, you will still need detailed records of your earnings and losses.

These records will allow you to see whether your personal training side hustle is financially successful or not. Without a record, you could be losing a significant amount of money without even realizing it.

Additionally, a personal trainer with a side hustle must also record their finances for tax purposes at the end of the year.

In order to keep track of your transactions be sure to pay close attention to your bank statements throughout each month. Alternatively, you can use online payment records to monitor your income and expenses, with apps such as:

- PayPal
- Stripe
- Monzo

I must stress the importance of keeping a note of every purchase or sale that you make in order to fill your tax self assessment. Failure to provide accurate information regarding your personal trainer side hustle can lead to serious financial consequences, such as owing a large lump sum of money.

Don't Be Afraid to Ask For Help

Taking the plunge and starting a personal training side hustle can feel somewhat overwhelming, especially if this is your first time working outside of contracted employment.

However, things don't need to be as scary or stressful as they may appear, and you should always reach out if you're struggling with any aspect of your side hustle.

If you find yourself in this position repeatedly it may be worth seeking out a mentor for support.

Tips for Growing Your Personal Training Side Hustle

Becoming a personal trainer as a side hustle doesn't stop once you've earned your qualifications and gained a few clients. If you're interested in finding further success, then you should be looking to expand upon your existing business model.

This section is dedicated to just that, and will provide you with helpful tips, all of which have been specifically chosen to assist in your personal training side hustle.

Create General Fitness and Nutrition Plans

In addition to providing tailored training for your clients, it may be worthwhile ensuring that your side hustle features general guides for others to purchase.

In this sense, you can use your PT and specialist sports nutritionist qualifications to create a general guide, featuring workouts and diet plans that are more holistically focused on health and fitness, rather than the individual's specific goals.

This method of distribution would expand your side hustle to a section of clients that would otherwise go untapped.

Remember, not everyone is comfortable with the idea of a personal trainer reviewing their workout or diet. For this group, being able to follow a premade template is the ideal solution to this issue, allowing them to work at their own pace.

This can be an easy source of revenue that takes very little effort on your behalf to create, just be sure to post regular updates in order to ensure these clients have updated plans to work off.

Create an On-Demand Workout Membership Website

If you launched your personal training side hustle out of a love for teaching sessions then why not consider launching your own on-demand workout website.

This is popular method of modern day personal training which I often associate with popular brands, including:

- Peloton
- Daily Burn
- FIIT
- Zwift

However, please keep in mind that the vast majority of brands lack the personable interaction that comes along with running your own business.

You can differentiate from all of these aforementioned corporations by creating an on-demand membership program that clients have a direct involvement with.

By doing this clients will feel a greater sense of comradery, and are more likely to want to stay subscribed or even purchase additional features.

Some ways that you can involve clients include:

- Taking polls to see what workouts they want to see
- Engaging in regular chats and discussions
- Offering consultations to subscribed members
- Providing incentives to stay signed up, such as branded merchandise

Much like the previous point, creating an on-demand service can help to expand your personal training side hustle to newer audiences.

For example, the clients who subscribe for this may not live in your local area or country, and would therefore be otherwise unable to attend your sessions.

You can make a real difference with an on-demand subscription service dedicated to your teachings.

Offer Different Services from Competitors

This point was touched upon within the previous section, but it bears repeating, as it's vitally important to identify gaps within the local market in order to provide services that your competitors are not.

I previously discussed how qualifications such as Sports Massage Therapy could benefit your clients following an intense workout. Certain individuals may be attracted to the unique offer of a sports massage to help them unwind after a workout.

But what about during the training session itself?

Specialized workout qualifications such as a Yoga Teaching Diploma could see you significantly grow and expand your client base, in order to reach an audience that could otherwise be missed or overlooked.

For example, yoga is incredibly popular in its own right, and attracts a different subsection compared to regular gym-based workouts.

These individuals may have otherwise ignored your offer of traditional personal training, but upon hearing you provide a yoga-based service may be more incentivized to sign up.

Appealing to different demographics of clients is vital in ensuring that your business thrives. Yoga was just a given example, but if you can identify an under-represented group within your local fitness community be sure to capitalize on it as soon as possible.

Start Researching Ways to Market and Advertise Your Side Hustle

Online marketing and advertising can seem incredibly intimidating at first, but I guarantee that the idea is far more stressful than the actual process.

As a personal trainer, you should be looking to advertise your side hustle across various platforms such as Google, Instagram, and Facebook.

Millions of potential clients use these platforms on an hourly basis, seeing your ad just once could prompt them to sign up for training, so make a good impression.

Some good news is that advertising on Google My Business is completely free.

Google My Business, also referred to as Google Snap Map, highlights local businesses that show up when searching for a specific service.

For example, when clients search 'personal trainers near me', they could potentially be greeted with your side hustle, granted that you rank within the local 3 pack.

Alternatively, Facebook and Instagram can be set up in order to fulfill a number of purposes such as:

- Get more engagement such as likes, shares and comments on a post
- Drive more targeted visitors to your website
- Get more Direct Messages from prospective clients
- Get more enquiries on Facebook or Instagram itself.

Facebook in particular holds a large amount of personal data, meaning that you can optimize your ads on the site to hit a very specific target audience. For example, if you're looking to target female clients, ages 30-60 who want to lose weight then that is easily achievable.

Marketing and advertising are just processes which seem complicated in theory, but can be implemented by any trainer, regardless of experience in order to grow their side hustle.

Become an Affiliate For a Fitness and Health-Related Product

Once you have established your personal training side hustle you will naturally find gear and products that are perfectly suited for your sessions.

If you find yourself routinely using and favoring specific health and fitness brands or related products, then it may be worth investigating whether you can become an affiliate for it.

You may be reading this section and rolling your eyes, believing this process to be something that only Instagram influencers are able to attain. However, many fitness companies use affiliate schemes to ensure that personal trainers refer their clients to their business.

The following fitness brands have affiliate programs that you can sign up as part of your side hustle as a personal trainer:

- **Reebok** - 7% Commission rate

- **Fitbit** - 3% Commission rate

- **Argos** - 2% Commission rate

- **BeachBody** - 15% Commission rate

- **Amazon** - 10-12% Commission rate

These affiliate schemes are easy to sign up for and could help to grow your personal training side hustle with the aid of extra money every month.

Become a Sponsored Personal Trainer

Similarly, if you'd like to reach the heights of fitness influencers you should research ways that could lead you to becoming a sponsored personal trainer.

In order for this to occur you're going to need to produce high-quality social media content that will attract the attention of brands. This in itself is a challenge that will help to grow your personal training side hustle but can be achieved by creating the following content:

- Competition giveaways
- Motivational quotes
- Diet and nutrition advice
- Fitness and modeling tips
- Themed content for holidays or special events
- Collaborations with other trainers
- Memes

The biggest piece of advice I can give to maximize the potential of growing your clientele is to use hashtags, specifically 10 per post. Some can be general such as 'fitness' or 'personal training', whilst others should be niche and reference what the post is discussing.

As you begin to amass a following you may begin to encounter brands offering to sponsor you in one way or another.

If you find yourself in this type of situation you may receive offers of the following types of sponsorships:

- **One-off Reciprocal Sponsorship** - This may not be a financial sponsorship but can see you receiving something you want off a brand such as equipment or gear. In this instance, a personal trainer will usually receive the product in return for advertising on their socials. They will then be given a bespoke discount code that their followers can use in order to purchase the same product. However, this will only be temporary and will expire after a set date.

- **Continuous Reciprocal Sponsorship** - With the ever-growing power of social media brands are always looking to develop a long-standing relationship with fitness influencers. If you fall under this category, a brand will usually refer to you as a 'brand ambassador', who will promote their products all year around. As with the one-off sponsorship, no fees are typically exchanged, but the service or products you receive will be continuous for as long as you remain an ambassador.

- **Retention Sponsorship** - In this instance, a brand will pay a retention fee, in order to ensure that the fitness influencer promotes their product on a regular basis.

- **Reward Sponsorship** - A reward sponsorship is granted following the success of a specific marketing campaign. A fitness influencer will promote a service or brand and will receive a payment based on the sales that their followers generate.

Ultimately, I can say that sponsorship can help to significantly grow your side hustle as it has the potential to be incredibly lucrative. While this might seem unattainable when initially beginning your business, it can be achieved through hard work and dedication.

Implementing any of these recommendations can see your side hustle grow in numbers. Once again I would like to advise the importance of taking time to develop your client base, as this is something that will happen gradually over time rather than instantaneously overnight.

Benefits of Starting a Personal Training Side Hustle

Throughout this chapter, I have discussed the many ways that becoming a personal trainer as a side hustle can lead you to personal satisfaction and financial success.

However, there are several other benefits to pursuing this career path, all of which will be fully explored within this dedicated section.

You Can Choose When and Where You Work

One of the most appealing aspects of becoming a personal trainer as a side hustle is that you get to personally decide when you work, and where you work.

Whether you want to be in a contracted role with several hours allocated every week, or a mobile personal trainer who works on a freelance schedule is entirely up to you. This helps to alleviate any stress and negative feelings that may otherwise appear when taking on a second job.

If you can't personally take the stress of clocking into a second job following the end of an intense shift then you simply don't have to. Make your schedule and approach to training work for you, as this should be a fulfilling role not a stressful one.

Have a Positive Effect on People's Lives

In your current full-time job role, you may have no direct interaction with customers or clients, and may feel that you don't positively impact upon their lives.

However, by following personal training as a side job you can directly see how your influence is affecting the lives of others.

If you speak to any qualified personal trainer, they'll agree that one of the most rewarding aspects of the role is the positive effect you can have on the lives of others.

Whether you're helping a client to reach personal goals, recover from an injury, or simply being there for them, you can make a difference and positive impact on their lives within this role.

Therefore, I can say that this positive impact won't only benefit your clients, it can help improve your life too.

Think how good you will feel by helping someone to obtain a fitness goal that they've been pursuing for years.

Adds Variety To Your Life

Feeling unfulfilled within your full-time role could negatively impact on your physical and mental health. It's easy to become caught up with the 'same-old-same-old', but a personal training side hustle can add a distinctly unique sense of variety to your life.

Regardless of what classes you teach, or services you offer, you can constantly change things up and avoid boredom and repetitivity whenever possible.

Are you becoming bored with teaching aerobics classes? Then why not switch it up and pursue HIIT training instead - you'll keep things exciting for you and your clients that way.

Unsatisfied with solely conducting regular personal training programs? Pursue another qualification and find a new area of interest such as yoga training.

Therefore, I can say that adding variety can not only benefit your life, but that of your clients too.

You can avoid some of the boredom we often associate with the same daily routine. With a personal training side hustle, you can really shape your own day and improve your happiness in the process.

Build a Side Business Without a Loss of Income

Launching a new career can be a somewhat risky financial decision. Leaving the safety and comfort of your regular full-time employment doesn't always pay off, and those who rush into the practice full-time may, unfortunately, suffer the consequences.

However, when deciding to pursue personal training as a side hustle, this fear is non-existent, as you don't have to instantly give up your primary source of income.

Instead, you can rely on your existing salary to support you, paying for bills and food while you pursue your fitness passion on the side.

If worse comes to worst and things sadly don't work out for your side hustle, then you won't be left with a mountain of debt or unpaid bills. The financial safety net provided by your full-time salary will be there to catch you and help you get back on your feet.

Alternatively, you may find your side hustle to be more financially rewarding than you initially expected, which could prompt you to take on the role full-time.

Potential To Go Full-Time

Finally, I can say that another benefit of this role is that it has the potential to grow from a side hustle into a full-time career.

Taking the plunge to fully enter the fitness industry can be intimidating, especially if you're already comfortable within your existing full-time role.

Therefore, launching this side hustle could be viewed as testing the waters, allowing you to determine whether it's something you wish to pursue even further.

However, it is worth noting that operating in a full-time personal trainer position is very different from a side hustle.

Just be sure to make the right decision for yourself, and not rush into things without a detailed business plan in place.

PERSONAL TRAINING OLDER CLIENTS

The older generation are an often-neglected target audience when it comes to personal training. But in fact, personal training older adults is a lucrative niche with an ever-growing demand.

I love old people! They're witty, sarcastic, rude, sweet, loving, and wise all at the same time. They deserve far more than we give them. Seniors enjoy staying active, and retiring allows them to cancel the majority of their plans. Consider this: we spend a lot of our time at work, and when we're not there, we spend time getting ready for work, winding down from work, and even attending work events.

Take that away, and you'll find yourself with plenty of free time. Seniors, like children, can benefit from walks in the park. Especially in nursing homes. An events coordinator may work in a nursing home. You can have them walk around the facility or gather in a common area for low-impact workouts.

Seniors are straightforward and easy to work with. Because they enjoy dancing, a simple dance/workout routine would be ideal.

In this chapter, I've got some top tips for personal training seniors, so you can start taking on clients from this demographic.

What Do We Mean By 'Older' Clients In Fitness?

Before we get into some tips for personal training older clients, let's establish what exactly we mean by 'older' clients.

So, at what age are you classed as 'older'?

Unfortunately, there is no concrete answer. But in healthcare, for example, geriatric care is typically for those over 65 years of age. This is the age also typically used when referring to older adults in the context of fitness.

For the purposes of this book, we will use the terms 'older adults', 'seniors' and 'mature' interchangeably to refer to clients over 65.

However, you don't need to be overly strict about this number. For example, if you have a client who is 60, you can still apply my tips on personal training for older clients, even if there are a couple of years difference.

According to the NHS physical activity guideline, older adults should do some form of light activity every day. Light activity can be anything from a walk around the park to standing up and sitting down.

They also recommend at least 150 minutes of moderate activity (e.g. cycling, walking, tennis) or 75 minutes of vigorous activity if you are already active (e.g. aerobics, swimming, hiking).

Just like people of all ages, many seniors will get a personal trainer to help them reach these exercise goals.

One major misconception about mature clients in the fitness industry is that older means weaker or less fit - this is not always true.

The older generation are indeed more likely to have health conditions or injuries that affect their strength or restrict their physical movement. But equally, young people can have these issues too.

In fact, an older adult can be just as if not more physically fit and healthy than someone half their age.

You need to have an open mind when personal training mature clients. But at the same time, you should of course be aware of their age and adapt your sessions accordingly. But do not underestimate them.

Steps to Personal Training Older Clients

Start with an assessment

Before you start personal training an older client, it is essential to conduct an initial assessment with them.

An initial assessment is a chance to assess your client's current fitness level and identify any injuries they may have. This will then help you determine their goals and create a tailored and effective program for them.

This usually takes place wherever you will be training your client- whether in the gym or in their home, and should last between 30 minutes and an hour.

Here are 3 things I recommend doing during your first assessment with an older client:

1. Make them feel comfortable

This first session is a great time to establish a positive and supportive relationship with your client and ease any nerves they may have.

This is particularly important when personal training older adults, as they may be feeling apprehensive about returning to training after a break or after an injury, for example.

Keep in mind that many older clients may not have trained for a while, and some may have never set foot in a gym in their life.

You can make your client feel comfortable by starting with some general small talk, before you go on to talking about fitness. This will help them ease any nerves and help establish a rapport between you both, and make them more receptive when you come to discuss training.

2. Find out about their health history

This is important when training anyone, but particularly when working with the elderly.

You should take notes on any past injuries, health issues and previous exercise experience. These factors will help determine the kind of exercises you include in their program, as you may need to make modifications to some exercises to accommodate for these things.

For example, someone with a lifetime of exercise experience will be able to do a very different level of program compared to someone who has hardly ever exercised before, or a client who has only recently recovered from a long term injury.

You may also want to carry out a postural assessment as part of this. This will give a good indication of their muscular structure, alignment and the range of motion in their joints- the latter of which is particularly important when personal training mature clients.

3. Establish goals

This initial assessment is also a great time to establish what your client's exercise goals are.

In general, older adult's goals will more likely be functional, rather than aesthetic focused.

For example, many younger clients may be more interested in getting a certain physique, such as a six-pack, or building their glutes.

But older clients may be more interested in achievements that will improve their day to day, such as bending down to pick things up or being able to walk to the shop.

I recommend using the SMART fitness goals criteria to ensure that your goals are Specific, Measurable, Attainable, Relevant and Time-Bound. For example, a SMART fitness goal for an older client could be:

To be able to touch your toes in 4 months time, by improving hip and hamstring flexibility.

Having a clear goal in mind will help you create a program that is truly tailored to your client's needs. You can also keep referring back to it throughout the program to monitor their progress and keep them motivated.

Build up strength slowly

When personal training seniors, some PTs can be scared to use things like dumbbells and kettlebells with their clients. But being older does not necessarily mean weaker.

In fact, strength training is particularly important for seniors, as strength and muscle mass can decline a lot faster in older age.

However, this doesn't mean you should go straight to the squat rack with an older client.

Instead, adapt the type of strength training you would typically do with a client, perhaps by working at a lower intensity and focusing more on resistance than lifting heavy.

For example, you should work on basic movements such as a bodyweight squat, focusing on increasing range of motion and encouraging them to use good form before adding any weight.

When they are ready to add weight, start small and increase in smaller increments than you would usually.

Fractional weight plates (i.e. 0.25 and 0.5kg) are a great way to do this. Over the weeks, months or years, these small increments will all add up.

Avoid extreme/ high-intensity exercises

When personal training older adults, you should generally avoid more 'extreme' exercises.

This can include explosive cardio exercises such as burpees, sprints and box jumps.

Weighted explosive exercises include things like the clean and press or kettlebell swings can also be too much for elderly clients, as they require a high level of stability and balance as well as strength.

Extreme HIIT workouts are also generally not advised when it comes to personal training for older clients. Although the general principles of interval training are beneficial for everyone, you should reduce the intensity for more mature clients.

Instead of high-intensity workouts, focus instead on flexibility and mobility, using slow and controlled movements.

Don't neglect cardio

Although you should generally avoid extreme movements like sprints, this doesn't mean that you should completely avoid cardio when working with seniors.

There are lots of benefits of cardio, particularly for seniors. For example, it strengthens the respiratory and circulatory systems, which is especially beneficial for older adults as these systems can naturally become weaker with age.

However, you may need to adapt the type of cardio you do. For example, older adults are more likely to have balance issues, so running on a treadmill may not be a good idea.

A better choice would therefore be to use more supportive machines, such as the seated bike.

Walking is also one of the best forms of cardio you can use when personal training seniors. This could be done on a treadmill, or you could encourage your client to walk more in their daily life outside the gym.

Warm up

Warming up and cooling down is always important, but especially when personal training older adults.

Some benefits of warming up are:

- **Increases body temperature.** This makes more oxygen to flow to the muscles, which will allow them to contract and relax more easily during exercise. This is particularly beneficial for older adults who may be more sedentary during the rest of their day, so their muscles will need time to warm up.

- **Reduces the risk of injury.** Warming up the muscles before exercising helps increase their elasticity, which reduces the risk of overstraining them. This is particularly important for older clients to do as they are generally at a greater risk of injury.

- **Helps them mentally prepare for the session ahead.** Warming up before launching into the bulk of your session also allows your client to mentally prepare for exercise. It also allows them to settle into the gym environment, as well as increasing focus and concentration!

- **Increases range of motion.** Older clients will typically have a smaller range of motion in their joints, such as the ankles, shoulders and knees. Warming up will help these joints reach their maximum range of motion before exercising.

Any kind of stretching you do before a workout should be dynamic, rather than static. In other words, the stretches involve movement, rather than holding a stretch for a long period of time.

Some examples of warm-ups you could do with your older clients are:

- Walking or jogging on the spot (30 seconds to 1 minute)
- Shoulder rolls (20 each direction)
- Neck rolls (10-15 reps)
- Ankle rolls (10 each side)
- Side stretches (10 each side)
- Standing quad stretch holding on

The whole warm up should last around 10 minutes, but may be more or less depending on the ability of your client and the length of your session.

Cool down

As well as warming up before your session, you should include a cool down afterwards.

This allows your client's muscles to slowly relax again after being used, and allows the heart rate to slow back down to a normal pace.

This is particularly important for older clients, as abruptly ending a workout could cause dizziness or a sudden decline in blood pressure and blood sugar levels, which is of course dangerous.

Stretching the muscles whilst they are still warm after exercise will also help prevent injury and reduce muscle soreness and the likeliness of cramp.

Cool-down exercises for older adults should be easy on the joints, so avoid any inversions such as the downward dog.

Some good example of cool-down exercises for seniors are:

- Chest stretch

- Standing quad stretch

- Seated hamstring stretch- these hamstring stretches for lower back pain are particularly beneficial for older adults.

- Corpse pose (lying down on the floor)

Like a warm-up, a cool-down should be around 10 minutes long. But again, this depends on how long your session is.

Focus on flexibility

As well as strength and cardio, you should also focus on building flexibility.

There are so many benefits of flexibility training for everyone, but particularly when personal training mature clients.

This is because as we age, we are more likely to lose muscle tone, skin elasticity and bone density. Tendons and joints get stiffer too, which all results in reduced flexibility.

The benefits of flexibility training for older clients include:

- Decreases risk of injuries such as fractures and strains
- Improves ability to carry out daily functional tasks (such as bending down to pick things up)
- Can delay the onset of health issues such as arthritis and diabetes
- Improves posture
- Increases mobility and range of motion in joints
- Improves circulation

When doing flexibility exercises with older clients, never force a stretch and always take things slowly. Keep stretches simple and even seated if possible, for example a seated overhead side stretch would be a suitable option.

If you do give them a standing stretch, such as a standing quad stretch, make sure to have the client hold on to something like the wall or the side of a chair.

You should also encourage them to keep a slow and steady breath through a stretch, and never lock out joints.

Be clear with your instructions

Strong communication skills are one of the most important skills of a personal trainer, and this is especially the case with older clients.

When working through an exercise with a mature client, you may need to give even more detailed prompts than you usually would.

This is because as I have mentioned, they may not have done these kinds of exercises before, or at least not for a long time.

For example, you may have younger and more experienced clients who understand what to do when you say, 'engage your core'.

But if an older client has never heard this term before, you will need to give more prompts to help them understand how exactly to do this.

You may also need to explain exactly what the core is, so that they can have a better mind-to-muscle connection. You should therefore be prepared to break down exercises in more detail than you may be used to.

As well as good communication skills, this requires patience - a skill which we will explore in more detail later in this chapter.

Keep exercises close to the floor

A good tip for personal training the elderly is to keep exercises close to the floor. In other words, use exercises where they have a low center of gravity.

This is simply because the older you get, the more balance can become an issue, increasing the risk of falling.

So when offering personal training for older clients, stick to exercises that are close to the ground or involve two feet on the floor at all times, such as:

- Squats
- Mat-based ab exercises such as planks, crunches, bicycle twists and leg raises
- Push-ups
- Bicep curls (standing or seated)

Since balance deteriorates with age, you could also counter this by including some exercises designed to strengthen their balance.

However, remember to modify any balance exercises to make them safer for older clients who are more at risk of falling.

For example, you could work up to a single leg balance by getting them to hold on to the wall or a chair first.

You should also always spot older clients, more so than you would with others, even during bodyweight exercises. Again, this is because there is a higher risk of them losing balance and falling.

Think about where and when you train

When personal training seniors, you may need to think more about where and when you hold your sessions, and if need be, adapt to the needs of your client.

For example, a loud, busy gym setting at peak times may not be the best time or place for an older client who is hard of hearing.

Plus, in a busy gym there is more risk of bumping into people or equipment.

If you are training an older client in a gym, you may therefore want to opt for off-peak times.

Many older clients may even ask if your sessions can be held in their homes, particularly if they have mobility issues that restrict them from leaving the house.

Training clients in the comfort of their own home has tons of benefits for both you and your clients.

Focus on the hips

Hip pain is a notorious problem that comes with old age, so it is important to include plenty of hip-strengthening exercises when personal training older adults.

Weak hip muscles can make it difficult for seniors to perform everyday tasks such as walking, going up and down stairs, and bending down.

However, before doing any hip exercises with an older client, make sure that you have established whether they have any existing hip problems or not, as they may be under guidance from their doctors as to the kinds of movements they can do.

Some hip exercises that are particularly beneficial for seniors are:

- Glute bridge
- Hip circles
- Seated marching

* Standing hip abduction

Unilateral exercises

A bilateral movement is when the limbs on both sides of your body are used at the same time, whereas a unilateral movement is when each limb works independently.

For example, a barbell curl requires you to use both arms to move one weight, making it a bilateral exercise. An example of a unilateral movement would be a single arm bicep curl using a dumbbell.

Most people have a dominant side of the body that they feel is stronger. When performing bilateral exercises, the dominant side will naturally take on more of the stress of the movement - often without the client even realizing.

Whether intentional or not, overusing a dominant side can lead to muscle imbalances. Over time, imbalances can increase the risk of injury or pain - particularly in seniors.

Including unilateral exercises when personal training older clients will help counter these imbalances by building strength in both sides of the body.

Unilateral exercises also encourage a greater mind-to-muscle connection (i.e. actively engaging muscles rather than passively moving), which will help improve strength and flexibility.

Plus, unilateral exercises can help strengthen the abdominal muscles, as engaging the core is what keeps the body stable and aids the movement.

Since just one side of the body is used at a time, unilateral exercises can also help improve balance.

Unilateral exercises to use with your older clients are basically anything that involves movement from a single limb, such as:

- Single leg drops
- Lunges
- Single-arm bicep curls
- Step-ups

Skills Required For Personal Training Older Clients

The skills required to be a personal trainer for older clients are very similar to the skills of a general personal trainer, however, there are some skills which are particularly important when working with this demographic.

Patience

When personal training older clients, you will need to be more patient than you may normally be.

You should be prepared for smaller achievements and perhaps slower progress, especially if your client has an injury or has not exercised for many years.

If you're training a client who has never been in a gym setting before, you'll probably have to take more time to explain how to use certain equipment than you would with a client who is used to being in a gym.

You may also find that older clients do not pick things up as quickly as your younger clients. To accommodate for this, it is a good idea to do more demonstrations yourself to show them how to do it.

It is also a good idea to do the exercises at the same time as the clients so that they can mirror your form.

Flexible

Offering personal training for older adults might mean that you need to be more flexible with your training program than you would with other clients.

This is because elderly clients are more likely to have more health issues or injuries that affect their ability to do certain exercises.

You should therefore be willing to change and adapt exercises as you go, not just after the first assessment.

For example, during a session you may notice that your client has very tight hamstrings, making it difficult for them to perform exercises such as deadlifts.

Instead of just removing the exercise from their program, you could instead adapt it by including exercises to help improve hamstring flexibility- such as a standing hamstring stretch. You could also include other hamstring strengthening exercises, such as heel raises.

Over time, their hamstrings should get stronger and more flexible, and they may be able to work their way up to doing a deadlift with proper form.

Having the flexibility to adapt your training program like this shows that you are dedicated to helping your client make progress!

Motivational

Being a motivating role model is always a key role of a personal trainer, but it is particularly important when it comes to personal training seniors.

You may find that your older clients lack confidence, especially if they have not exercised for a long time or are not familiar with being in a gym environment.

It is therefore up to you to give them the confidence boost they need!

The best way to do this is simply by giving them words of encouragement throughout the sessions. Giving them positive feedback after an exercise is also a good way to reassure them and increase their confidence.

As well as making them feel confident and comfortable, don't forget to challenge them! Setting challenges and goals, whether for the session or the whole program, is highly motivating.

For example, at the start of a session, you could set them the challenge of doing 8 reps of squats without stopping. By giving them a definitive target to work towards, this will motivate them throughout the session.

Tracking their progress is also important when personal training older adults.

This could mean tracking their physical progress (e.g. body measurements, weight, before and after photos), or whether they have experienced any mental benefits (e.g. checking in with how they are feeling).

All of these methods help your client see their progress, which will motivate them to carry on and stay interested in training.

Respectful

As I mentioned earlier in this chapter, there is a misconception surrounding older adults in fitness that they are weaker and slower. This can sometimes lead personal trainers to underestimate their older client's ability, and treat them differently to other clients.

Instead, when personal training seniors, treat them with the same respect that you would with any other client - despite any health issues or problems they may have.

For example, you may need to adapt your communication to accommodate a client who is hard of hearing.

But this should simply mean raising your volume and making sure that your pronunciation is clear, rather than adopting a patronizing or belittling tone of voice.

Remember that as a personal trainer, you are there to build confidence and motivate your clients, not bring them down!

Building a good relationship with your older clients is not only important on a moral level, but it will also ultimately help you to retain clients. An older client in particular is much more likely to stick with a personal trainer that they know respects them.

How To Become A Personal Trainer For Older Clients

If you're still with me at this point, you're probably fairly interested in becoming a personal trainer for older clients. So, here's how you can achieve exactly that.

The good news is that if you're already a qualified personal trainer, there is nothing stopping you from taking on older clients.

You do not need any special qualifications to train older adults.

However, if you want to specialize in offering personal training for mature clients, there are some additional qualifications you can take which may benefit your career prospects.

Having further qualifications will improve your own knowledge and allow you to offer a more specialized service. This benefits you by making you feel more confident in your abilities, and also benefits the client since they'll be getting a better service.

Specialized qualifications are also useful when it comes to attracting new clients and tapping into a niche, such as personal training for older clients.

By completing an advanced course related to the needs of elderly clients, you can market yourself as an 'expert' in the area which will make it easier for you to attract clients from that specific demographic.

I will discuss marketing yourself as a personal trainer for older clients later in this section, but for now here are some additional qualifications that could benefit your career.

Lower Back Pain Management Courses

Lower back pain is a very common problem amongst the senior population, so having this qualification means that you can confidently take on and train clients with these issues.

A Level 4 Lower Back Pain Management course teaches students key skills such as how to identify posture issues, muscle imbalances, and different types of back pain.

On completion of the course, you'll know how to create and deliver specialized programs to promote recovery and aid rehabilitation for such issues.

Nutrition Qualifications

Other specialist courses such as a Level 4 Advanced Sports Nutrition can also be beneficial when working with any clients, including the elderly.

Having this qualification not only means that you can offer nutritional advice to your clients, but also gives you a more in-depth knowledge of the relationship between food and exercise.

This will also allow you to deliver a more specialized service to your older clients, helping them get better results and allowing you to charge a little extra for your sessions.

Getting Qualified in Exercise Referral

A popular route of career progression for personal trainers who work with older clients is to become an exercise referral specialist.

Exercise referral is the process of a medical or health professional referring a patient to a fitness programme, with the aim to improve their health through exercise.

Some conditions and illnesses that clients could be living with include:

- Diabetes

- Arthritis

- Lower back pain

- Osteoporosis

- High cholesterol

- COPD

Many of the clients who are referred to an exercise referral specialist are older adults with such health conditions.

Once you have some experience working as a personal trainer for older adults, it's likely that you'll be familiar with working with these kinds of clients.

Studying an exercise referral course will allow you to offer an even more specialized service to such clients by equipping you with the skills and knowledge needed to be able to help clients recover from illnesses and cope with chronic health issues.

You may have come across some course providers who offer courses specifically for training senior clients. But as I have said, you do not need a specific qualification to work with older clients.

If you simply follow the tips in this section and take any additional qualifications to further your knowledge, you can absolutely become a successful personal trainer for older clients.

Benefits Of Personal Training Older Clients

As this article has shown, there are lots of benefits of older clients getting a personal trainer. But you may now be wondering, what's in it for me?

Here are some great benefits of personal training older clients that you may not have thought of:

Helps you stand out from other PTs

Compared to other demographics, there are relatively not many personal trainers who specialize in training older clients.

This is a huge benefit for you, as it means that you can stand out as a personal trainer in this particular niche.

By choosing a fairly unexplored avenue of personal training to go down, you will have less competition from other PTs, and therefore a higher chance of gaining clients!.

For example, an older adult is much more likely to choose a personal trainer who specializes in training older clients, over a more general personal trainer.

Clients want a personal trainer who they know will be able to create a program that is as tailored to their individual needs as possible.

This is particularly true for older adults, as they may have specific injuries to consider, for example. They will therefore want a personal trainer with experience in training older clients who may have encountered their injury before.

As such, an older adult is much more likely to choose a personal trainer who specializes in training older clients, over a more general personal trainer with no experience working with seniors.

You can charge more for your services

Since you will be a 'specialist' in personal training mature clients, you can justify charging more for your services.

This is because people are more likely to pay a higher price for a specialist service, compared to a generic service that may not be tailored to their needs.

For example, since there are not many personal trainers that specialize in older clients out there, you will be in a higher demand. You will be seen as a specialist, so people will be happy to pay a higher price for your services.

Over time, as you start to build a reputation as a personal trainer who specializes in older clients, you can start to increase your prices even further!

You can develop more targeted marketing materials

If you are a specialist personal trainer for older clients, you can create more targeted marketing materials.

The Importance of Marketing Your Fitness Business to Seniors

Seniors refer to the demographic of people from 50 and above. Unfortunately, most personal trainers overlook this demographic, assuming they don't want to be active. But this is not the reality. Lots of seniors want to be active and maintain healthy lifestyles.

So, if you have not been marketing your personal training services to this demographic, you could be missing out on a steady source of revenue for your fitness facility or club. If you are still not convinced, here are some more reasons why you should be marketing personal training services to senior citizens.

Seniors are More Committed

People over 50 understand the great benefits of regular exercise. Also, they exercise regularly to manage or reduce chronic pain, reduce the risks of falls and injuries, improve sleep quality, and reduce muscle atrophy.

Hence, unlike younger people, their motivation to exercise regularly goes beyond aesthetics. As you may expect, seniors will be more committed to working out regularly compared to younger people. Consequently, you can expect them to continue renewing their gym memberships.

They Have the Money to Spend on Fitness

According to Market Watch, seniors contributed to approximately 40% of the U.S economy's GDP in 2018. And this number is gradually growing, as more people join this demographic.

And with great retirement benefits, mortgages paid off, no dependents to drain their finances and with homes that have acquired considerable value, seniors have money to spend on things they care about. And this includes their health and well-being.

So, if your personal training marketing strategies have been solely focused on young people, it's time to re-strategize and start marketing to older adults too.

More Publicity for Your Gym

As much as you will be holding most of your personal training for seniors inside your gym, they also provide an opportunity for your fitness center to become more visible in your local community.

For instance, you can provide on-site fitness programs in a nearby assisted-living facility. And while you may offer these services for free or at a heavily discounted price, the event will be a source of good publicity for your fitness center.

And with good publicity, there's a high chance your gym will attract even more clients, who may have never heard about your services before that event.

Seniors are a Rapidly Growing Market

According to the United States Census Bureau, approximately 115 million Americans were 50 and older in 2019, representing at least a third of the population.

Over the next 10 years, this demographic is expected to reach around 132 million, according to a report published by the AARP. And this translates to more spending power for this age group.

In contrast, there are approximately 45 million people between the age of 20 and 30, which is usually the main target group for most fitness centers. At the same time, this number is expected to remain stable over the next couple of years.

Hence, focusing your personal training advertising strategies on people over 50 offers your personal training business a huge market, not only today but in the years to come. Simply, this age demographic provides a huge earning potential today, and the future is also promising.

Higher Retention Rate

Older adults usually face social isolation as the years go by. Hence, it becomes increasingly important for people within this demographic to maintain social connections.

The problem is, it's not always easy for them to find suitable activities for their age, which can help them to maintain social connections.

And this is where fitness centers come in. By providing a place for seniors to stay fit, socialize, interact and integrate into the community, you can help to minimize the social isolation they usually face.

You can also engage them in activities like group workout sessions or social support. And by having a thriving senior community in your fitness center, you can rest assured the retention rates will be higher.

How to Market to Senior Citizens

As earlier mentioned, the personal training advertising strategies you will use with younger people may not work with older adults. So, how do you convince this demographic to join your fitness center? Here are some tips on how to market to seniors.

Define Your Target Audience

The demographic for older adults is quite diverse. Hence, when you create your personal training advertising campaigns for seniors, you should not target them as one large group.

Instead, you need to clearly define your target group within this demographic. For instance, you can opt to target men or women, diseased or healthy, fit or frail, retired or still working.

You also need to go a step further and narrow down your target client to their marital status, economic status, hobbies and interests, the charities they support and where they live.

Narrowing down to the type of older adult that you intend to target will help you to specifically come up with personal training ads that effectively speak to them.

Establish Yourself as a Fitness Expert

Older adults tend to respect those who have specialized in their areas of expertise. Hence, by positioning yourself as a fitness expert, you will become their go-to person on matters related to fitness. And this presents more opportunities for you to convince them to join your gym.

So, how can you establish yourself as a fitness expert? Well, you can do so by publishing fitness books, writing fitness articles, giving presentations at fitness events, or even appearing in local news.

Focus on Selling them What they Want

Older adults join fitness centers to improve their overall health and fitness so that they can continue enjoying life. And while they may want to lose some weight, attaining the physique of a 20-something year model is not what they are after.

Therefore, whenever you are designing your personal trainer ads, you should focus on addressing the key health and fitness challenges this demographic is facing. By using this approach, you will find it easier to convince them to join your personal training program.

Seniors are still pretty old school so advertising I would probably go with fliers that you can hang or slip under their doors. Be sure to list the price. You do not want to trick them. I would also encourage the family to participate on my flier. It can be quality time and it helps them to see that their parents are staying healthy. Don't get me wrong, seniors are able to get online and I've noticed that they love Facebook of all the social medias so posting your flier there may be beneficial. It's free so I don't see it hurting anything.

Once you've gotten your group established, begin to get feedback. Your members will tell you what they like and dislike. I suggest making the adjustments and watch them advertise for you. You will no longer need flyers or Facebook and you may even have to do more than one session to fit them all.

How to Retain Older Personal Training Clients

By following the above personal training marketing and advertising tips, you will manage to bring some older adults to your workout class. But, bringing them through the door is one thing. You will also need to work on retaining them. After all, there may be other fitness centers in your area targeting the same clients.

So, how do you make sure that the older personal training clients that you've just acquired don't cancel their memberships?

Here are some tips:

Avoid Loud Music

Loud music can prevent a senior from hearing your instructions clearly. As a result, you may be forced to raise your voice.

And while this may not be a problem if you are training a younger person, older adults may not be comfortable with you shouting at them. Hence, if you have to shout instructions to them, then that may not be the ideal environment for personal training older adults.

If you have to play music, you should keep the volume low. Also, make sure you select tracks that are appropriate for this age group. You can even ask for their recommendations and then shuffle the tracks as they train.

Create Time and Space for Them

We all hate working out in crowded fitness clubs. And, it's going to be even worse for older adults.

Older adults have a fear of getting knocked over and falling. So, if your gym is jam-packed, there's a high chance they will not be there for long.

Also, a considerable number of them use hearing aids. So, if your fitness center is jam-packed, it will affect their ability to distinguish sounds and voices. Again, this may heighten their anxiety while increasing their risk of getting injured.

To prevent these issues, you should have dedicated workout sessions for older adults. This way, they can comfortably enjoy their workout session without the anxiety and fear that comes with a crowded gym.

Keep the Instructions Simple

Training older clients can be a bit tricky compared to younger personal training clients. But, regardless of the approach that you take, make sure you keep your instructions simple and clear.

Doing so will help to eliminate confusion, making it easier for them to follow your instructions.

And if they can follow your instructions clearly, it will be easier for them to attain their health and fitness goals.

Older adults deserve personal training services, just like any other demographic. However, most gyms, fitness clubs and personal trainers don't market their services to this demographic, meaning they are mostly left out. But as earlier mentioned, personal training older clients can be a source of steady income for your fitness business. Besides, it can also be extremely rewarding, as you help them to regain or maintain the ability to be fit, active and independent.

START A FITNESS YOUTUBE CHANNEL

So, you've been pondering over how to start a fitness YouTube channel for a while now but you're not sure where to start. Does the mere thought of it make you feel overwhelmed? Well, I get it. You're not alone.

Here's the thing:

YouTube has transformed the way the fitness industry operates today. It is growing exponentially and poses a wonderful opportunity for anyone trying to make a living out of fitness videos.

The good thing? You don't need celebrity trainers, expensive cameras, or professional crews to create fitness videos. It's all about your zest for leading a healthier lifestyle and the **unique content** you bring to the table to inspire others.

Whether you're a personal trainer trying to reach potential clients, or a fitness vlogger trying to hit more subscribers, or a beginner who's all set to start a fitness

YouTube channel, or a fitness brand who's trying to grow your business, video marketing is essential.

And if you think about it, fitness people prefer learning from videos rather than going through lengthy blog posts.

Stick with me till the end, as I am going to guide you to do everything right.

Why Should You Create Fitness Videos on YouTube

They say that a picture is worth a thousand words.

But ever wondered how much is a video worth?

Well, a whole lot! Don't just take my word for it, do your research and let the numbers speak for itself.

The fitness industry is evolving continuously, and over the years, I have seen it grow from a mere nothing to a multi-billion dollar conglomeration, which has become vital to millions of people worldwide.

The global fitness industry witnessed tremendous growth in the past few years and is estimated to be more than $96 billion. With so many enthusiasts and influencers, the YouTube fitness community grew enormously—to the extent that Youtube reported that their "home workout" content category inclined by 515%.

So it's loud and clear

Interest in watching fitness videos is increasing year on year, and YouTube, being at the forefront with a huge global reach than other video platforms, just can't be ignored.

Fitness plus Video gives a dynamic combination. Videos are the ideal platform for storytelling and it isn't a surprise why fitness studios, personal trainers, and enthusiasts worldwide are leveraging it as a key lead generation channel.

While I have given you enough reasons to start a fitness channel on YouTube, here are a few more to inspire you:

- Lets you tap into a wider audience

- Helps leverage the home workout crowd

- Increases brand awareness

- It's easier to show than to describe

- Search engines value video content

- Enables you to create fitness content that helps people

- Earn revenue via YouTube ads, brand sponsorships, and affiliate programs

While the benefits outweigh the downsides, it's important to note that starting a fitness vlog or channel takes effort and time. And you need to have a lot of patience because the process isn't overnight.

How to Start a Fitness YouTube Channel

Committing to creating YouTube content is easier said than done. But it's half the battle won if you have a proper plan in hand.

Here's a step-by-step guide to help you learn how to start a fitness YouTube channel:

Define the goals of your YouTube channel

Ask yourself these questions:

- Why am I creating this fitness YouTube channel?

- What outcomes do I want from my fitness YouTube channel?

- How different will my fitness YouTube channel be from the rest?

- What are the other ways to monetize my fitness videos besides YouTube?

The answer to these questions will give you a complete picture of what you want to achieve from your YouTube channel. Then, set benchmarks to accomplish these goals either quarterly or half-early. Make sure to keep your goals realistic and achievable.

Know your target audience

After your goals are in place, understand the audience you are creating the fitness video content for. This will help you produce video content attuned to what they want to engage with.

Speaking of which, there are 4 key things you should know about your audience:

- **Demographics:** This is your audience's age, gender, and location. This data will help you create videos in a language and format that caters to them.

- **Psychographics:** These are characteristics that drive audience behavior. For instance, their values, lifestyle, motivations, aspirations, and insecurities. This data will help you understand the various ways to connect with the audience emotionally.

- **Online behavior:** This gives you an overview of what your audience prefers to watch for entertainment. It includes insights into the type of channels they like to subscribe to, social media sites they are on, and their average spending time. This data will help you create content that best engages them.

- **Offline behavior:** This includes your audience's purchase behavior, hobbies, habits, work status, and where they prefer spending their time at. These data insights will help you create content that evokes emotions in them.

While the above is true, go a little further in understanding better about your audience to create fitness content that they will find useful.

In order to do so, ask yourself these questions:

- What are the real pain points that your target audience face?
- How much is too much to pay for fitness training online?
- What factors put you off from other fitness programs that you have tried?
- What's their average income?
- What's their fitness routine look like?
- What other interests do they have?

Knowing and understanding your audience sets the stage for you to create video content that will resonate better and entice more people to convert to your paid programs.

Find out what your competitors are doing

Keep an eye on other fitness YouTubers and the type of videos they are creating. This will help you come up with unique content ideas.

- **Watch videos in the fitness niche:** Observe what type of fitness videos (long-form, short-form, tips, tutorials, etc.) creators are making.
- **Subscribe to your competitors' fitness channels:** Note the frequency of videos your competitors create.
- **Delve into their comments sections:** Browse the comments to gauge what people think about your competitors' videos. Try to understand what they are lacking and jot down the things that could have been better.

- **Look at their video views:** Find out which videos have the highest views and engagement levels.

All of this will help influence your own content schedule and what your content plan should look like.

Validate your content ideas

Before taking any steps to create a fitness YouTube channel, it's vital to validate your content ideas. This is pretty simple and straightforward to do.

Ask yourself these questions:

- Is there a good demand for what you will be creating?

- What are they asking for if there's an existing audience for the niche?

- What could you do better than your competitors?

Conduct keyword research to verify how many people are looking for things relevant to your content idea. Here are some handy tools to help you with keyword research: Google Keyword Planner, SemRush, or AHREFS.

List the type of fitness videos you want to create

While you're excited to start your fitness YouTube channel, it's important to note that it's a wide niche, and there's a lot you can cover, but you cannot do it all. So think of the type of fitness videos you want to create.

Keep your target audience in mind and what they enjoy watching or engaging with on YouTube.

Here are some fitness video ideas to help you get started:

- Home workout
- Diet and nutrition
- Yoga & meditation
- Fitness challenges
- Health and fitness tips
- Healthy food and recipes
- Fitness or weight loss journeys
- Daily exercise or workout routines

- Reviews of home gym equipment and accessories
- Reviews of protein powders and fitness supplements

Create your video content calendar

Once you know the type of fitness videos you want to create, the next step is to have a detailed calendar that includes a proper publishing schedule.

- Outline when, what, and how frequently you will be uploading videos to your channel
- Pick 10-12 topics your audience will love watching online and create a proper publishing calendar around them.
- Pick a day and make that your "publishing day" and stick to it because consistency is the key.

Create your YouTube account

All you need is a Google account (or Gmail) to set up your YouTube channel. Have a Google account under the name of your fitness channel.

Once that's done, here's what you need to do:

- Sign-in to YouTube via your brand's Gmail.

- Navigate to your account page on YouTube and click create a new channel.

- Customize the dashboard. Update your homepage banner by uploading a nice photo (max size: 4MB) that signifies your brand.

- Edit your profile and complete the sections under the About & Description tabs.

- Add links to your blogs, websites, and other social media accounts.

Shoot your fitness videos

You don't need fancy DSLRs or high-end cameras to shoot. You can invest in them later on when your viewership grows.

Here is some basic video equipment to help you get started:

- **Smartphone:** Your phone is more than enough to shoot your videos. But make sure to invest in a tripod, though.

- **Lighting:** Videos recorded in a well-lit space look pleasing, high-quality, and professional. Invest in a good quality ring light to cast off those shadows and keep your footage inviting.

- **Hardware:** Though mobile apps help edit videos on your phone, a computer is highly preferred because it gives you enough storage space to save your edited videos and have them as a backup just in case something goes wrong with your channel.

Edit and upload your fitness videos

Unlike Instagram and Facebook Live, YouTube videos require editing. You don't have to learn complex video editing tools for this. You have plenty of video editors online that can edit your footage in no time. Most of these tools have free trials and are cost-effective.

You don't need complex software or special skills to edit your fitness videos. You can do that faster and without breaking a sweat through online video editors.

Share and promote your videos on social media

Lastly, it's time to share and promote your videos. You can do this in multiple ways. Send it to a verified email list, use your social media platforms, or embed your YouTube links in blogs to reach a wider audience.

If you have made up your mind, creating a roadmap or a business plan for your fitness YouTube channel is the next step. It will keep your short-term and long-term objectives in sync while ensuring you stay 100% focused on the purpose of starting one.

Your business plan doesn't have to be detailed. It should be basic enough to let you know you're on track.

YouTube Common Terms

You don't have to be a tech guru to launch a branded fitness channel on YouTube. Nonetheless, here are some common terms, in simple language, that you'll want to familiarize yourself with before diving into creating a YouTube channel.

- **Audience retention**: describes your channel's ability to retain its audience.

- **Avatar**: also known as your channel artwork; it's the square space with a custom image of your choosing that represents your channel throughout YouTube.

- **Branding watermark**: a brand image, or logo, that appears in the bottom right corner of your video that allows a viewer to subscribe to your channel by clicking the watermark.

- **Bulletin**: messages that channel owners can send to the channel's subscribers via the subscribers' feed.

- **Call to Action (CTA)**: clickable phrases or images that request the audience to perform a task, such as click a link, complete a form, or subscribe.

- **Channel authority**: your channel's total watch time (in minutes) that affects your channel's YouTube ranking.

- **Channel header**: graphic displayed at the top of your channel homepage

- **Channel homepage**: the front or feature page of your YouTube channel that includes your channel header, community tab, video tab, and channel trailer.

- **Closed caption (CC)**: captions and subtitles that are closed in a colored background for readability.

- **Community tab**: the channel owner can post messages, digital content, and polls which the channel's subscribers will see in their feeds.

- **Copyright**: "In many countries, when a person creates an original work that is fixed in a physical medium, they automatically own copyright to the work. As the copyright owner, they have the exclusive right to use the work. Most of the time, only the copyright owner can say whether someone else has permissions to use the work." (Visit YouTube's Help Center for more details regarding copyright and rights management.)

- **End-slate**: a graphic that is strategically placed at the end of a video with a CTA.

- **Evergreen videos**: videos that cover non-time-sensitive topics—avoid news and current events—and are great ways to grow your channel because the content remains relevant for years.

- **Featured content**: you can arrange your channel's playlist to feature recent or popular videos on the channel's homepage.

- **Metadata**: text that describes a video in the form of titles, tags, and a description.

- **Monetization**: the authorization of ads (Google Adsense) throughout your videos.

- **Paid content**: videos that are pay-wall protected, keeping the content visible only to paid subscribers.

- **Sub for sub or collab**: when channel owners follow each other's channels for the purpose of growth.

- **Tags**: relevant keyword or key phrase descriptions that are added to a video prior to uploading that make the video more discoverable on search engines.

- **Thumbnail**: a custom image and simple text that represents your video when it appears in YouTube searches.

- **Video card**: text (website or link) that is displayed in the top right corner while your video is playing.

BECOME A DANCE FITNESS INSTRUCTOR

Now for my favorite workout of all time, the dancing. So this really works. My friend and I did it, we had fun and we lost weight. It just really works. How I would propose that you accomplish this is to first go online to YouTube or whatever and seek for the line dances, the trending line dances. That seems like the Cha cha slide, the wobble, even the electric slide. Learn them, get them down packed. Everybody is doing these dances, so if you're able to teach them to others in a fun workout atmosphere, they're going to come.

Like they say, if you create it, they will come. If this is a real statement, I would again propose going to the park or someplace free and taking your Bluetooth speaker and just vibe out. Just have fun with it. Lead everybody step by step, teach them what they're supposed to do, and then run through the dance a few times. I would each week have them come back, learn more, and maybe let this class last for about 6 weeks.

This one you're going to be able to get a little more money for because again, people love to dance. You can even do this one with the senior citizens. You can simply just come up with a fun dance routine if you like to dance. It doesn't necessarily have to be the Slides Or Line dances.

If you know you enjoy dancing and you know some interesting routines, then put them together. Put it out on your flier, put it out on Eventbrite that you are going to be leading or teaching new popular dances. Get the word out and watch them come. For this one, I would charge $10 a session or like I indicated earlier, if you have it last for six weeks, you may just say, you know, 50 bucks for the whole six weeks and you'll meet. Maybe twice a week or once a week. Whatever works for you.

Like I said before, dancing is my favorite, I love to dance and I know this actually works in losing weight. So, I'll be offering suggestions on how to be a dance fitness instructor and also how to lead a fun filled dance workout class in this chapter.

How to Become a Dance Instructor

Moving towards a new career or class concept armed with rhythm and a desire to make people feel amazing, can seem like a dream come true for many.

Here I would like to share my top 5 tips on how to get started with becoming a dance fitness instructor:

Find your vibe

There are so many different styles of dance and dance fitness as well as a whole host of teaching methods. If you have a passion for a certain style of dance or music then this will start to pave the way towards a certain brand or creating your own class around a specific theme.

There really is something for everyone in dance fitness – for instructors and participants, which is great because we are all so different with what we love and are truly passionate about helping people stay active.

Connect with your clients and potential clients

It might sound basic, but what is your market really looking for? This will help shape how you construct your class if you are going freestyle. If they are after something upbeat with a higher intensity then that will let you know what bpm or movement patterns you might look at. Do they already have experience in dancing? Could this be the first fitness dance class they have ever done? Then that will change what you might add in too. The same goes for branded concepts. Choose something that fits you and your target market will make it a lot easier to sell as well as to connect with.

Make sure you have the right qualifications

Ensure that whatever qualifications you have extend to the concept you wish to cover. The first port of call for someone with no fitness or dance background would be to look at a group exercise qualification. Being qualified in the style of class you want to teach will also help you to pick up cover work at a gym or studio which will help you hit the ground running.

Reach out to local instructors

If you are looking to teach but you have no experience, why not attend a variety of classes whilst you work out what it is you truly love. Let the instructor know that you're intending to train up and they will no doubt be able to point you in the direction of other places to go locally or centers to reach out to that might need extra cover.

Think outside of the box

If you're looking for cover work, then sure, it makes sense to offer a class that's popular in your local area. But if it's your own class that you're looking for, perhaps it would be better to stand out in a busy market than offer the same style or concept. There is something magical about not being afraid to be yourself and teaching a class that makes you feel confident and your clients will feel exactly the same when they connect with you.

Tips for Planning a Dance Class

I have been to my fair share of bad classes (haven't we all) and it's particularly infuriating to have paid your valuable money to take part, only to realize five minutes in that you could probably teach the class better yourself.

Here are my top ten tips for how to plan a class (particularly an open, adult class; but most of the points are transferable to a number of settings).

Here goes:

Introduction

The first thing to do is speak to your class. Introduce yourself, the theme of the session, what you'll be doing and so on. A group of people in the know will be much more confident than if they have no idea of what they'll be doing for the next hour. Always take time to talk.

Never start with static stretches

Never, never, never do static stretches at the start of a class. This is dance 101 but you'd be surprised how many times I've walked into a studio to be told to start stretching straight away. Do you want to injure people? I should sincerely hope not.

Create the right vibe

Create the right vibe for the movement you're about to explore. This can be done by your choice of music, providing context for the genre (see point one) and the way you use your voice. E.g, nobody will be able to embody the Dancehall energy if you put on Latin music, use a soothing voice, ask us to stretch straight away and get us to do generic cardio as a way to warm up. Which leads me nicely on to the next point.

Introduce key movements

Always introduce key movements that you plan to use later on in the session, in the warm up. This will give your participants the opportunity to become familiar with movements ahead of time and reaffirms the confidence mentioned in point one. It's also a good way for you to see how many in the group find your movements challenging in comparison to those who seem really comfortable with them.

Endeavor to carry everyone along

No matter how your class is advertised, you will always have people of mixed abilities in the studio with you. Using descriptive language (similes, metaphors, adjectives) is a key tool to make your movements accessible to a range of abilities. If you can describe how a step should feel, or can liken it to a specific environment (e.g moving underwater) or sensation (e.g as if you have no bones in your body) it gives your participants something to visualize to help them make sense of your movement in their own body. You can only get so much from watching someone else demonstrate.

To accommodate further, always have simplified versions of your steps ready to pull out – particularly if you have movements that are fast, complicated or require a high level of strength or flexibility. Not everyone in the room will be able to execute your advanced choreography and they should not be made to feel bad because of it. (The other side of this is to also ensure you have a more progressive version of your steps to take into account those who may be highly-trained).

Ensure everyone feels valued

Leading on from this, to ensure everyone feels valued and as though they are doing a good job (which they will be!), each time you run the routine/sequence with the group, dance the advanced version(s) and then the standard version with them. Also avoid using the word 'easy'. Though it can be reassuring for some, it can be demotivating for others – use 'standard' or 'original' and 'advanced' to differentiate.

Keep an eye on the time

Keep an eye on the time. As ridiculous as this sounds, I am sure we've all been there when a teacher spends 40 mins on one section of a routine and then tries to teach the same amount of new material in the last 10 mins in order to 'finish it off'. Or worse, leaves only 5 mins in which you are expected to choreograph the next 16 counts yourself. Don't do this, instead, don't be afraid to deviate from your lesson plan. If it takes 40 mins for a group to learn five movements then leave it at that.

Don't rush them and try to teach your entire choreography because that's what you said to yourself you'd do. You'll have a messy group and everyone (including you) will go home feeling frustrated. It's far better to have a group of confident dancers performing 30 seconds of movement really well, than having a group of intimidated and confused dancers muddling their way through two minutes of material. If the creative element is a really important aspect to your class, introduce the task early on in the session. If they finish it with plenty of time, go back to teaching your choreography. Know your group, give them time and listen to them.

Don't single people out

Don't single people out/don't use negative reinforcement. Unless you are injured and cannot physically demonstrate a movement, don't ask the group to watch one of the participants as an example of what to do. Though it may feel uplifting to that one individual to be singled out in a positive way, the rest of the group may feel a) resentful that they won't be chosen or b) disengaged because they're not interested in a 'who does it best' contest.

Dance class is not bootcamp

Equally, if a group aren't picking up your movement, don't make them drop and give you twenty. This actually happened in an open class I was in. Seriously. *There are a number of problems with this but the main two are:*

a) Unless your class is part of an intensive training programme/academy, this level of discipline is not necessary and

b) This method of teaching is really excluding – what if your participants can't physically do a press-up/sit-up/squat jump or whatever it is you're making them do?

Not only will they feel rubbish that they can't do your movements properly (which they signed up to try), now they feel even worse because you've highlighted that 'deficiency' and given them another thing that they 'can't do' that they did not sign up for. Your class is not a bootcamp or a detention center, always be open and positive and you will get the best results. If they're not getting all of your choreography, go back to point eight.

Make time for your clients at the end of each session

Stick around at the end of your class. Quite often, participants want to have the opportunity to say thank you, ask questions, or generally just talk to you about their experience. Make time for them to do this and they're more likely to come back next week.

These are my top ten tips for planning a dance class.

The key thing to remember is that these people have paid to learn from you and should feel glad to be there. This isn't a showcase, no-one has signed up to take a class just to watch the teacher demonstrate or show off over and over again. They are there to learn.

Dance, of course, is centered around the body and people's individual body image's are complex things. In a dance class, you are asking people to move their bodies in new or unusual ways and you should always make space and time for them to do this in a positive and friendly environment. Confidence isn't built by tearing people down.

Tips for Creating a Fun Filled Dance Workout

Many group exercise instructors do not realize the full influence they can have on their students. In some cases, your class could be the best part of their day. But why? What about a group exercise class can turn that 30 or 60 minutes into the highlight of an entire day? The experience, especially if it is a fun one.

The experience involves how you as the instructor can make the participants think and feel. This isn't the super complex drill or choreography you worked diligently to teach perfectly. It's the fact that you remembered their name, or your playlist spoke to them, or maybe it was the endorphin-release you helped facilitate.

When teaching dance fitness classes, part of the experience is creating an environment where the participants do not feel self-conscious about their dance moves, but release, relax, and bust a move. We should be creating fun experiences so our class wants to come back regularly. So how can we do that and avoid becoming a strict dance –class instructor?

D (Direct Introductions)

Don't be the hidden DJ in the back of the club. As people enter, make sure you introduce yourself and try to take a few seconds to learn something about that person. Maybe they are new to the city, came with a regular participant, was a professional dancer, or have two left feet. Learn something so they feel like they have a friend automatically. This will alleviate some nerves and allow for the participant to relax a bit more.

A (Activities for partners or small groups)

Even if it is as simple as a cue to high five the person next to you at the end of a dance song, make your participants interact with each other. Partner games and activities are fun and can easily create a bond between people. Do you know of a song track your class loves? Have the entire class dance it together first, and then put them into small groups and have them dance together in their own little circle facing towards each other. Sure, the laughter and giggles will be abundant, but isn't that the point?

N (Navigate the Room)

Who says you have to stay up front the *entire* dance class? Those ladies on the back row may never want to stand front and center but I am sure they would booty bump with you once or twice. Obviously, you cannot stray from the front often, but move around your crowd when there is a chance in the choreography.

C (Coach, not Star)

Even in a dance class, you are a coach and not the superstar of the show. There are no spotlights, talent agents, or reasons that you should focus the class on your own skills. While sometimes we do get lost in the music and movement, make sure you are focusing on your participants. Are they having fun? Do they struggle with a certain movement, and if so, how can you break it down for them?

E (Exceptional Playlist)

There are so many music services and apps available for you as an instructor that it will make your head spin. From Spotify to Tempo Magic Pro, there are ways to create the perfect playlist for your class, your participants, and your style. But don't be stuck in a selfish rut; just because you don't like a genre, doesn't mean your class doesn't like it. Mix it up, find remixes or mash-ups, and be creative.

CONCLUSION

A side hustle isn't meant to be a burden or a drain. It should compliment your current commitments and enhance your situation, financially and emotionally. Whether a part time career in fitness is similar to your full time career or takes you into an entirely different field, you should enjoy the work and never find it a chore.

For a fitness side hustle to work, you need to schedule your commitments and make sure you aren't overdoing it. Personal training or delivering workouts to clients is all about giving; giving your time, patience, skills and stability to clients. It can take a lot of energy to be a successful PT and fitness professional, so you have to make sure you are looking after yourself. Get plenty of rest and watch out for the effects of burnout. When you find the right balance, a side hustle can be extremely rewarding and can put additional cash in your pocket.

To effectively add a fitness side hustle to your schedule, go easy at first – coach a few mornings or evenings a week (not every morning and/or evening). Factor in plenty of rest time while you get used to the swing of things.

Regardless of your approach, you must enjoy the process and not allow yourself to get overwhelmed. In time, you may even find that your side hustle is actually the career path you want to take full-time because leading a workout class doesn't have to be a side hustle, it has the potential to become a full time lucrative job.

I wish you the best!

About the Author

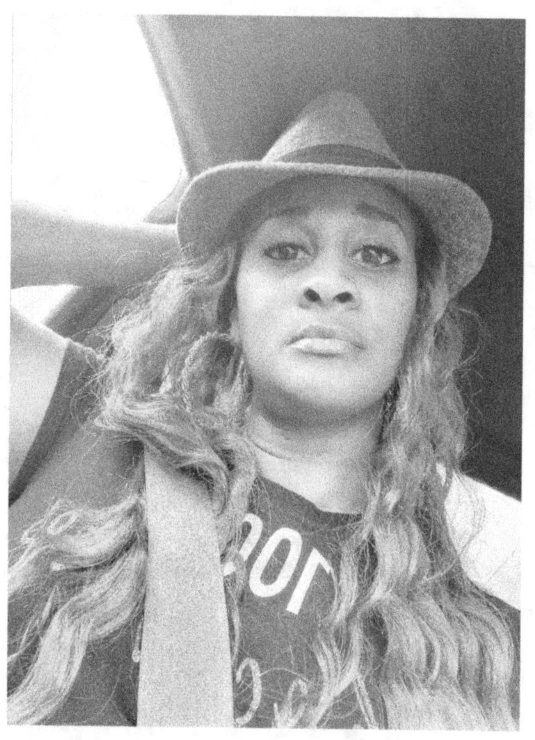

Hi, I'm Lovely the author. Thank you for taking time to read my advice piece. I'm grateful for your energy and for going on this ride with me. It's more than a blessing!

Life can be funny when it comes to dealing with humans, especially humans and money.

I'm a lover of love and laughter and find my inspiration in my mother and children. To grow up watching a single momma navigate life was truly an inspiration. Also watching my children navigate life from the very beginning inspires me.

My favorite part of writing is actually the story telling portion. I enjoy putting my spin on things and reliving the positive moments. Recapping lessons learned are also constant reminders that life is to be lived even in rough times.

I'm also a girly girl that lives in her feminine energy, good or bad. Sharing some of the private and possibly embarrassing moments wasn't the easiest.

I pray that conversations are had, situations are related to and people realize they are not alone when reading this book. I also pray for prosperity in all of your endeavors.

Thank you once again for reading my book and blessings all over your life.

~Lovely The Author

To contact me…
Email: lovelytheeauthor@gmail.com
Tik Tok: @Lovely the author
Insta: @ lovelytheauthor
Facebook: @ lovely theauthor
Youtube: lovely the author

9 798858 176701